MUSIC HEALS...

SUKANYA SENGUPTA, M.Sc., B.Ed.
Kolkata, West Bengal, India

and

ANUSHKA SENGUPTA, M.Sc.
Kolkata, West Bengal, India

2024

MUSIC HEALS...

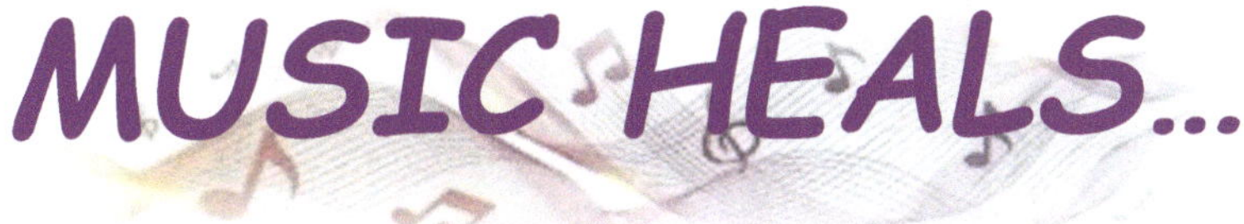

SUKANYA SENGUPTA, M.Sc., B.Ed.
Kolkata, West Bengal, India

and

ANUSHKA SENGUPTA, M.Sc.
Kolkata, West Bengal, India

Publisher

2024

ISBN No.

DOI.

Publisher

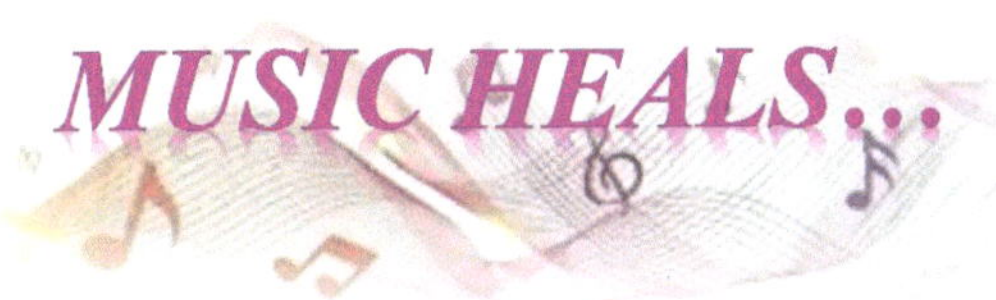

Content

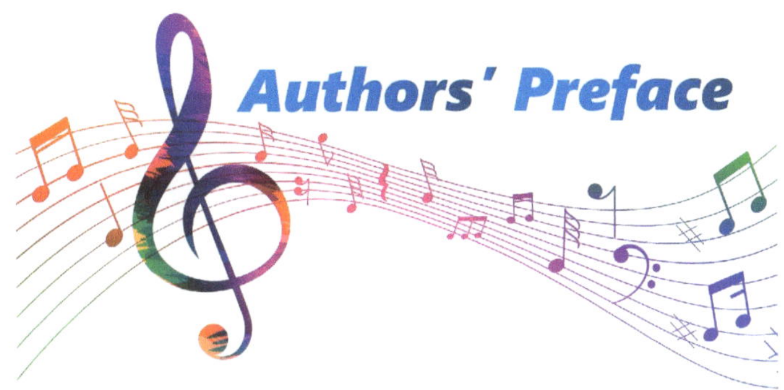

Authors' Preface

This book is not any syllabus oriented or related to any curriculum but just to get some extra information about Music. Actually more or less all of us are very fond of different kind of musics, but we have very limited knowledge about its proper utilization to make our life more happier and healthier. This book is written on such a topic that the reader from different field can understand the essence of the book and they can relate themselves to some extant.

Many new information hitherto unknown how to use this music medium to cure some diseases, which are very much common nowadays throughout the world.

The authors are intend to write the book on music for a novel purpose, so that relaxing entertaining music could serve as medicine vastly in future for human as well as plants and to explore about its magical power of healing besides amusement.

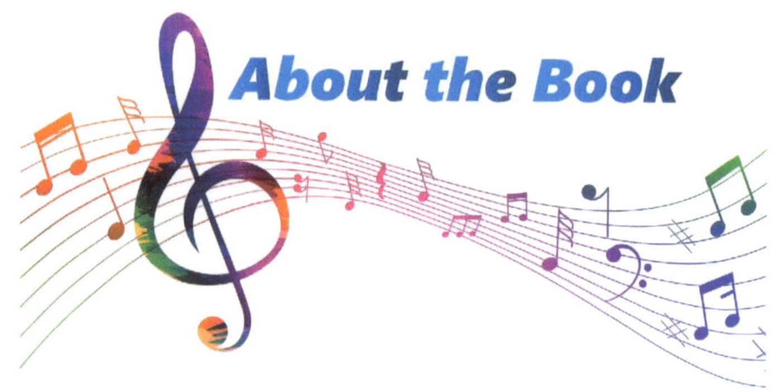

About the Book

This book is on music, is not as just a source of amusement but as the therapeutic or healing agent. Music is the sound where emotions can be expressed by the melody and rhythm along with beautiful harmony. Music has always a great impact on human in various ways, may be it cultural or psychological. Music has its own role on different age groups. Sometimes it is use to cure speech therapy, mental disorders, memory loss, etc.

Nowadays research shows how music can be used as the healing agent, which throws the light of hope of the new aspects of treatment.

Apart from human being music can heals the kingdom Plantae also. Music can influence the rate of productivity or yielding of plant.

But we should also now the limitation where to stop ourselves. Just like over dose of medicine, over exposure of music also may harms living beings.

About all this things authors have attempted to write the book to share their brief knowledge to society for its welfare and further utilization as no such book is available on this topic.

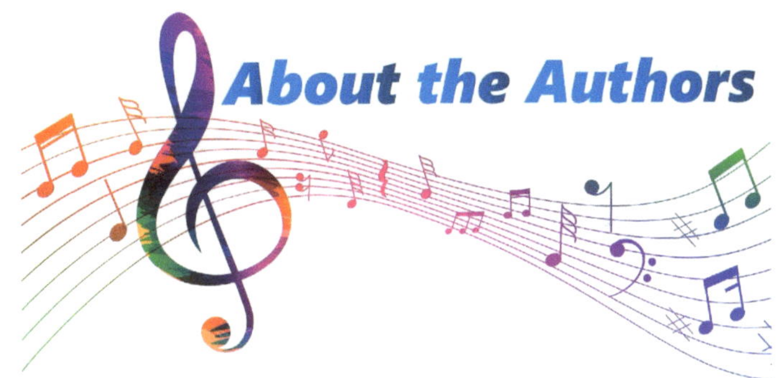

Sukanya Sengupta, M.Sc. (Botany), B.Ed., Biology teacher of a renowned school in Kolkata, with more than 7 years of teaching experience. Qualified GATE in LifeScience.

Anushka Sengupta, M.Sc., has initiated Ph.D. research work on Zoology (Acarology). Published three research papers in reputed journals along with one book published in more than 7 languages.

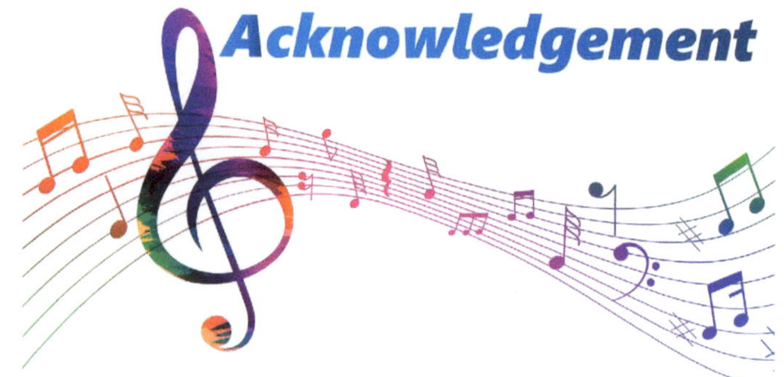

Acknowledgement

We want to express gratitude to our parents for supporting and encouraging us to write this document, as we have got support from every aspect of our lives from them.

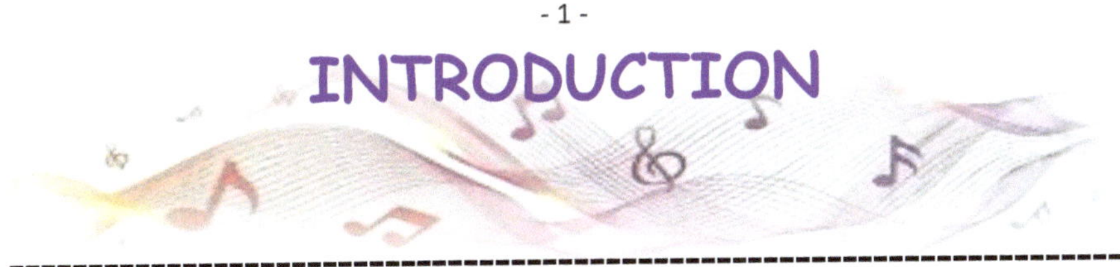

INTRODUCTION

"SOUND IS A NATURAL VEHICLE FOR LEARNING"

In this present condition, where the situation is going beyond our imagination, we need some magic which can heal our mental stress, and can give us some positive energy. "**MUSIC**" in such condition can act as one of the best medicine. It is not only relevant to this present scenario, but along with acting as a stress reliever, music has several important impact on human body as well as on plant body. Music increases our creativity, focus on work as well as IQ on other hand music enhances plant growth, flowering, fruiting, etc.

This document is on the usefulness of music. Where, we will get some brief knowledge about the importance of music as therapy, medicine for some diseases. Along with this music helps to secrete our happy hormone or good feel hormone called **Dopamine**.

Some survey on students proved that music can increase our memorizing capacity.

Finally we will know about the different frequencies especially about the healing frequency of music.

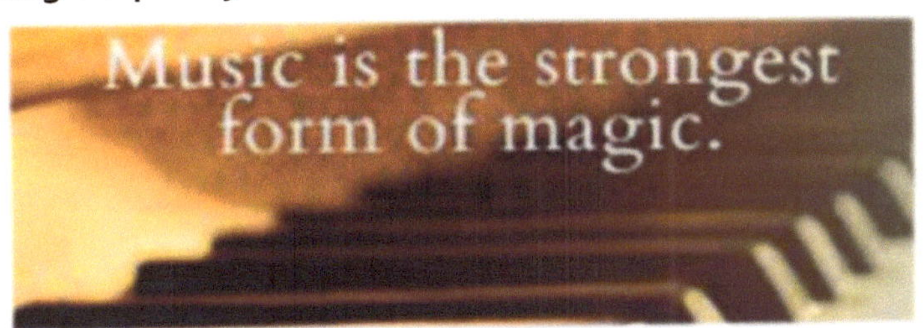

WHAT IS MUSIC?

Music is a creativity of sounds which signifies the present time, expressed some ideas as well as emotions. s

Sounds in single line called "**MELODY**",

Sounds in multiple lines called "**HARMONY**" and

Movements along with sounds is called "**RHYTHEM**" [Rhythm is associated with the movement, but not only the physical movement of the body but also the brain as well].

-----These are the most essential or main components of "MUSIC".

In some books, music is described as-

"Ah, music"..."A magic beyond all we do here".

-J. K. Rowling, Harry Potter and the Sorcerer's Stone.

"Music can produce one kind of pleasure which human nature can not do without."

-Confucius, The Book of Rites.

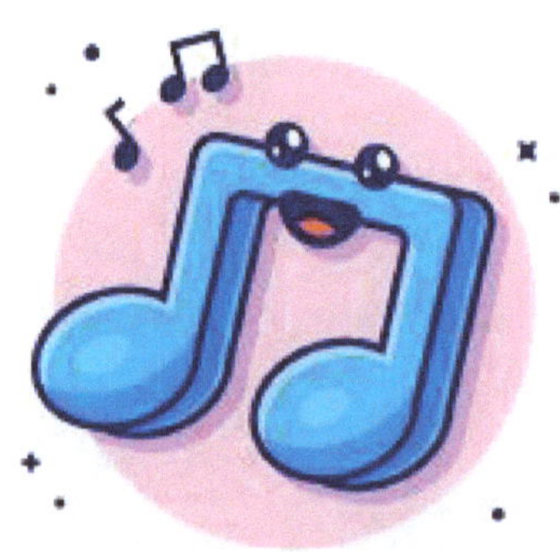

OVERALL IMPORTANCE OF MUSIC ON HUMAN BEING

➢ **MUSIC FOR HEALING:** Music can heal our brain, so automatically it heals our physical and emotional wounds. In ancient time both Aristotle and Plato used to prescribe music as a medicine of healing. The Greeks used to consider Apollo as the God or the king of Music and Healing.

➢ **MUSIC AND MEDICINES:** In hospitals now music therapy is considered as a major treatment for the patients of heart and brain, in case of speech therapy role of music is just like a magic.

➢ **MUSIC FOR THE ELDERLY:** Music acts as stress buster, it can overcome depressions also.

➢ **MUSIC FOR ADOLESCENTS:** Music can change emotional and depressed moods by counseling. The type of preferable music can predicts the behavior of adolescents.

➢ **MUSIC FOR MENTAL DISEASE:** Music helps to secrete more Dopamine [about 9% more] which can heal our brain as well as controls our movements by transferring signals from neuron to neuron and can increase memorization capacity. Music can be used to treat persons suffering with mental disease or illness irrespective of their age, it is very effective method for children having behavioral problems.

➤ **MUSIC AS COMMUNICATION:** Music is as natural among states, countries, and continents as speaking in a native tongue. Music can act as the form of communication without linguistic signs, conveying the intellectual, emotional and aesthetic meaning.

➤ **MUSIC THERAPY:** Based on several studies it has been observed that sometime music helps in recovery of the patients suffering from stroke, cerebral palsy, Parkinson's disease, traumatic brain injury etc. In the treatment of Alzheimer's disease music also having some influence. In case of epilepsy, music can normalize the electroencephalographic abnormalities.

➤ **MUSIC AND BRAIN:** Music can appear as an accompaniment in the gym or park during exercise, study shows that the synchronized music and exercise have potential physical benefits, where the "time of exhaustion" become 2/3 time longer than the usual time. Neuro-musicology, stating the relation between the nervous system and the people's interaction with music. Brain can group the sequences together and it can identify the relationships between the tones and sounds.

➤ **MUSIC CENTERS IN THE BRAIN:** According to neuroscience at least 18 areas of the human brain gets activated during listening to music, or performing music. There are many parts of the brain, that are used in perception and for comprehending music.

➤ **FOCUS AREAS FOR ASPECTS OF MUSIC:** Music have several specific focus areas based on different chords (consonant and dissonant) of music, activation of the music or harmony of the music i.e. different parts of the brain get activated and respond to different aspects of music. The brain can scan the listeners, who listen music only or imagining hearing it with the same area.

➢ MUSICIAN BRAINS: The neurological response differs between the musicians and non-musicians. According to the study by Christo Pantev's study it can be concluded that while listening to a piano playing the musicians use 25% more auditory parts of the left hemisphere of the brain than that of the non musicians. The musicians have 130% larger volume of auditory cortex than that of the non musicians.

➢ MUSIC LEARNING IN THE BRAIN: The musicians those before the age of 10, began to play music have different active regions of brain, sometimes having hyper development of some areas of brain.

➢ MUSIC AND INTELLIGENCE: Along with multiple use of music, skill of synchronization that occurs in the brain with musical influences that make human unique to any animal in the animal kingdom. Involvement with music leads to better memory, well developed intelligence, motivation power and also increase the thinking skills. It has opened a door of education which is always developing in the progress of student learning.

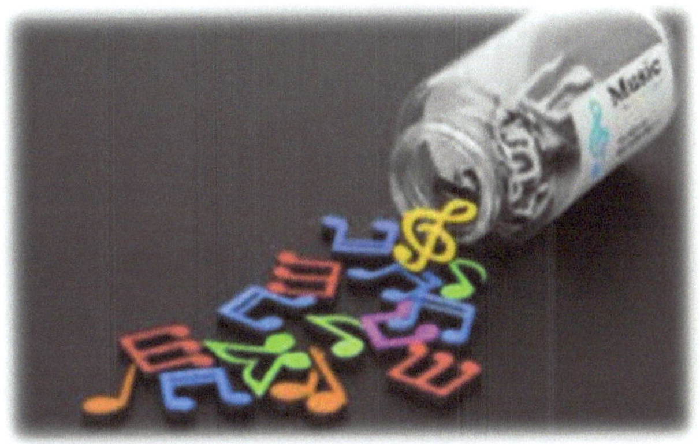

SURVEY AMONG STUDENTS

• METHOD-

A 10 question survey was done at Liberty University, among the students of several subjects like, music, biology, health, and from other variety of students. There were 57 males and 43 females under the survey. The questions were mainly based on study; they have listened to music or not, while studying, if yes, then the type of the music was also considered. Then the collected data were analyzed. 90% of the participants were between ages 17-22, 7% were between ages 23-25, and 3% were 26 and more.

• APPARATUS-

The survey was done with MCQs and one fill in the blank, designed by the author in Word Document.

• PROCEDURE-

The survey was done through almost one week, both in and outside of the class of the University. After collecting the data, those were analyzed using SPSS student Version 12.0 for the Windows.

• RESULT-

The ratio of the student was higher who listened to music while studying (55%). A good number of students reported that they listened to different types of music while studying, where as some were confined with only one or two types. Classical music was listened mostly (23%) by the students, then 20% used to listened to the Rock music and so on. The independent sample t-test were done, and the GPA showed [t(98)=- 1.182; p=240) no significance to those who used to listening to the music while studying. Then after collecting and analyzing the GPA of all the categories, the rap, hip-hop / Rock &Band , and Jazz showed lower GPA than the no music group.

• DISCUSSION-

The result of this survey showed no large effect on the student's performance if they listened to the music while studying. But, the regular exposure to rap and hip-hop have some negative impact on studies. The classical, easy listening music have positive effects on studies.

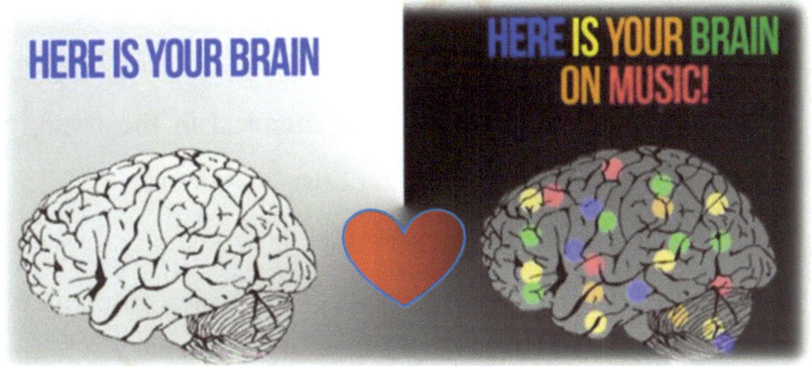

MUSIC ON PARKINSON'S DISEASE

➤ **WHAT IS PARKINSON'S DISEASE?**

Also known as "PARALYSIS AGITANS". Major cause is destruction of that portion of substantia nigra which are responsible neurons for dopamine secretion [Guyton and Hall Textbook Of medical Physiology, 12th edition, 693].

This disorder of Central Nervous System affects the movements often damages the nerve cells in brain that leads to secrete low levels of Dopamine.

❖ **IMPACT OF MUSIC ON PARKINSON'S DISEASE:-**

Music stimulates the release of a chemical in the brain, having an important role in setting good moods: DOPAMINE

According to the study, published in Nature Neuroscience a chemical (Dopamine) released as the response to music. Dopamine is such a chemical which increases by other stimulus like food and medicine. As per some study it is established that the transmission of dopamine is higher if the listener enjoys the music (the dopamine level can increase up to 9%). If the listener do not enjoys the music, less Dopamine secrets. For obtaining this data, to avoid any association with the lyrics (which may have different impact), only instrumental music is used in such cases. The data was observed through f-MRI.

MUSIC ON ALZHEIMER'S DISEASE

➢ WHAT IS ALZHEIMER'S DISEASE?

This is the premature ageing of the brain. Begins at mid-adult life and continuously progress to extreme loss of mental power at later old age. [Guyton and Hall Textbook Of Medical Physiology, 12th edition, 727] This disease can cause severe brain damage, degeneration of brain cell, destroying memories.

❖ IMPACT OF MUSIC ON ALZHEIMER'S DISEASE:-

A survey among Alzheimer's patients [The Effect of Music on the Human Body and Mind, Dawn Kent, 2006, 14] - A Russian composer Vissarion Shebalin studied when he suffered a stroke in 1953 and loss of his language capacities, mainly the abilities to speak and understand speech. But, music writing skills of Shebalin were remained same and Shebalin continued to compose music until his death in 1963. This study also reveals that Alzheimer's patients can recall words to familiar songs much better than spoken words or information. They can recall words of songs almost about 62% of the time, though they only remember spoken material about 37% of the time. Music helps in higher secretion of "FEEL GOOD HORMONES" like serotonin, prolactin, norepinephrine etc. which helps to reduce anxiety, stress etc. As music helps to increase memorizing capacity so it is broadly used to treat the Alzheimer's patients.

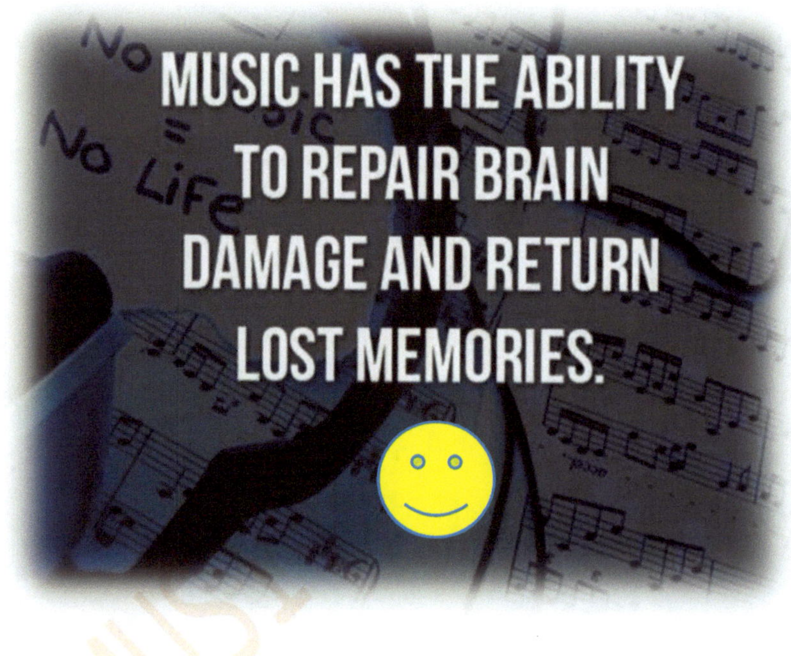
MUSIC HAS THE ABILITY
TO REPAIR BRAIN
DAMAGE AND RETURN
LOST MEMORIES.
No = Music
No Life

MUSIC ON DOPAMINE SECRETION

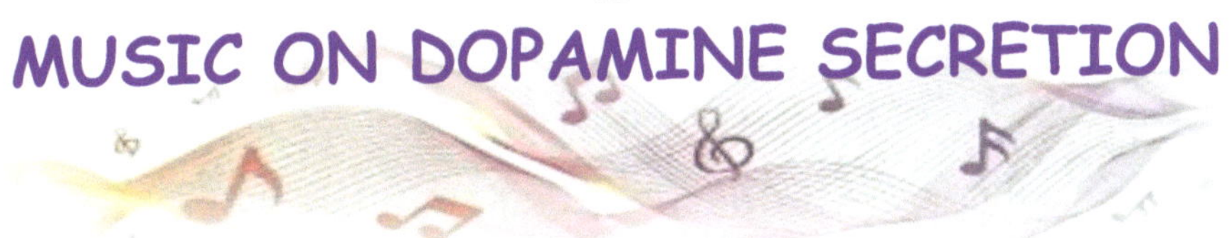

➤ WHAT IS DOPAMINE?

Dopamine is a one type of chemical neurotransmitter [from amino acid Tyrosine] , secreted by neurons of substantia nigra. Hydroxylation of dopamine can produce Norepinephrine [Guyton and Hall Textbook Of medical Physiology, 12th edition, 732]. It controls the physical and mental as well as emotions of human. It helps in body movement.

Dopamine is considered as one type of "FEEL GOOD" or "HAPPY" hormone. Along with enough sleeping, exercise, meditation; music can also boost up the secretion level of dopamine.

❖ Dopamine, casually linked with reward responses to music

According to a paper published on 28th January, 2019 in the 'National Academy of Science', it can be established that there can be "a link between the secretion of Dopamine (Neurotransmitter) and the reward responses to music".

As per the experiment, Dopamine transmission was pharmacologically manipulated showing the link among Dopamine, musical pleasure and motivation or encouragement. The precursor of Dopamine is Levodopa, which increase the hedonic experience i.e. (epicurean or indulgent experience) and motivation e.g. to buy a source of a song or to invest for a song. Risperidone, the antagonist of Dopamine leads to reduction of such indulgence.

From the above mentioned studies it has been observed that, pleasurable music induce the secretion of Dopamine. The stimulation of brain to the reward response related part of the brain can change the evaluation of music. This study throws the light in the fact that "Dopamine modulation can directly influence the people's experience of pleasure of music."

In the field of neurobiology and neurochemistry, the above mentioned result can form a bottom line or foundation of reward-responses to music (can be applied in disorders of reward and motivation in response to music).

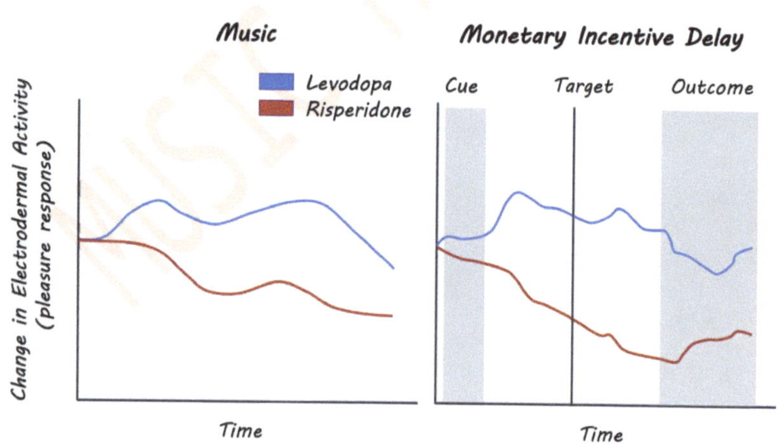

Listening to upbeat music can increase dopamine levels in the brain, which helps boost motivation and productivity.

SOLFEGGIO FREQUENCIES OF MUSIC FOR HEALING

Different frequencies of music can heals us at different ways. Solfeggio (Italian word) means SOL-FA a system where each notes of each scale has own unique syllable.

For example:-

174 Hz: REMOVES PAIN

285 Hz: INCREASES ENERGY

396 Hz: DECREASE FEAR AND GUILTNESS

432 Hz: SOOTHING, MAGICAL TONE OF NATURE

528 Hz: HELPS IN DNA REPAIRING

639 Hz: HELPS IN RELATIONSHIP HEALING

963 Hz: CONNECTS OUR SOUL WITH LIGHT AND SPIRIT.

❖ Effect of 528Hz music on the endocrine system and nervous system:

THE HEALING TYPE OF MUSIC

Based on another experiment, it was observed that music of 528Hz is a "Healing" type of music. Since, this frequency of music is directly related to DNA repairing so this frequency of music can also control our ageing process. That's why this frequency of music is very much important for human.

In an experimental procedure 9 people were treated with 528Hz and 440Hz (The tuning frequency for musical instruments) music on separate days. The salivary biomarkers of stress (cortisol, chromogranin, oxytocin) were measured in both the cases.

✓ The people who were treated with 528Hz music, showed the average level of cortisol and chromogranin was decreased significantly. Whereas, significant increase in oxytocin observed. ✓ When the people were treated with 440Hz no significant change in the salivary biomarkers were observed.

Based on a study (Sept,2018) it has been observed that if a person gets exposed to 528 Hz music the tension, anxiety and total mood difference gets reduced, whereas, in case of 440 Hz no such difference observed. After the experiment it can be concluded that only 5 minutes exposure to 528 Hz music has a strong stress reducing effect. High frequency music/sound can increase the synthesis of Dopamine and the activity of sympathetic nervous system can be suppressed, whereas, high frequency music can stimulate the activity of parasympathetic nervous system, resulting reduced stress.

Due to the vibrations of music biomolecules can rearrange their structure for better functions. Without proper vibration biomolecules can not work properly, but if we provide them the actual required frequency of music or vibration they will act the best.

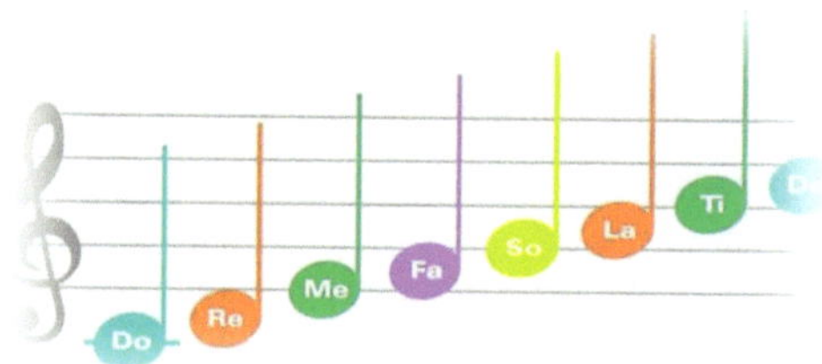

MUSIC ON PLANT GROWTH

A study in 1962, revealed that plant can grows 20% more faster when it exposed to classical music playing in flute, harmonium or violin (in presence of adequate basic needs for plant growth). Along with flowering, germination, fruiting of plants, classical and jazz music also activates plant defence hormone signaling pathway, helps to regulate secondary metabolism, activates immune system, enhances anti-oxidative molecule production, etc.

Researchers also proved that speaking nicely to plants can heal their wounds faster, supports their growth though loudness, shouting, harsh metal music are responsible for their stunting of growth and cause stress. In general, plants are more responsive in low level vibration around 115-250 Hz (this range is varies upon species to species).

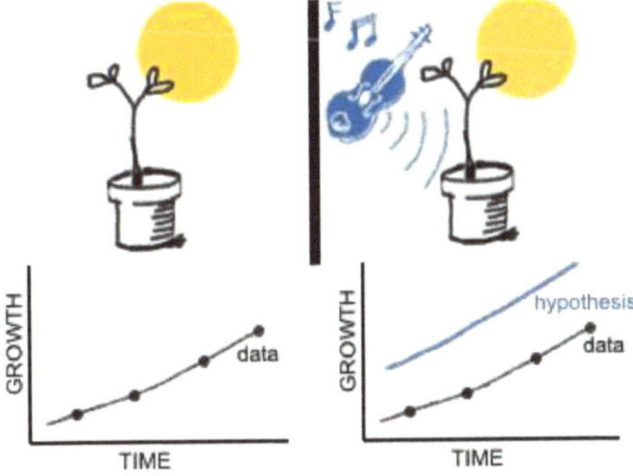

Music to stimulate plant growth

BEWARE AND BE AWARE

From this brief study on music, we can conclude that Music is not only acting as a source of amusement, but recent study shows that it can also act as an efficient/ potential method of therapy and it can stimulate particular cerebral circuit, having impact on neurological functions. The musical creativeness is to some extent associated with the psychopathological condition of a person. According to the study by the anthropologist and ethnologist it has been observed that music is a part of human characteristics over a thousand years. The different cognitive and emotional aspect / dimension of human life can be filled with positivity in association with music. Through several studies it has been observed that music can be beneficial for students' educational outcome. It has huge impact on social duties development, along with physical and psychological character development.

Though music is having several importance in our life, but long exposure to loud music or hard music may cause hearing loss. According to the scientists more than 15 minutes exposure can leads to severe damage. In fact a regular exposure to 110 decibel sounds for just one minute may result into permanent hearing loss. Use of headphones should also be controlled.

A loud rock concert can produce 120 dB. So, while getting exposed to such music we must keep the negative impact of the loud music in our mind. Even exposure to loud music during pregnancy may leads to a high risk of delivery of underweight and premature baby.

Evidences say that plants are also very sensitive to music, but other than classical, jazz music affects plant growth and development.

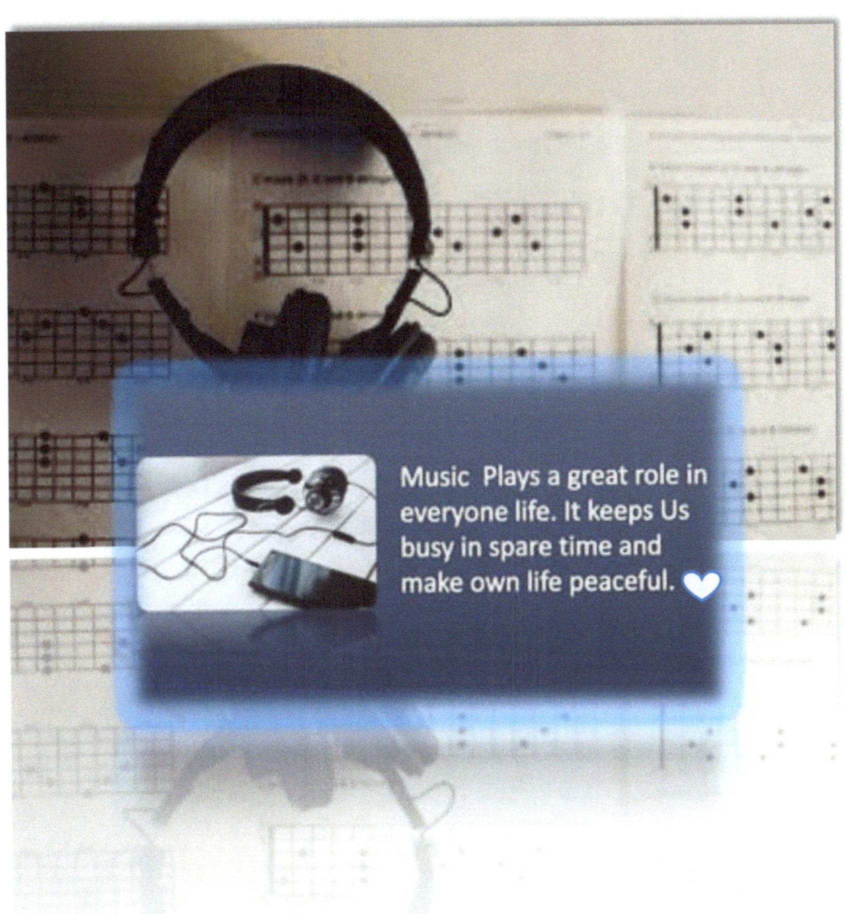

LIST OF SOURCES FOR FURTHER REFERENCES

- Hall, J. E. (2011). *Guyton and hall textbook of medical physiology* (12th ed.). W B Saunders.

- "The Effect of Music on the Human Body and Mind" by Dawn Kent (liberty.edu)

- "This is Your Brain on Music: The Study of Musical Influence on the Cog" by Allysa N. Lipsey (olemiss.edu)

- (PDF) The Essential Difference: The Truth About The Male And Female Brain (researchgate.net)

- How music affects the brain — University Affairs

- http://creativecommons.org/licenses/by-nc/4.0/

- http://dx.doi.org/10.1007/978-3-319-16999-6_2844-1

- https://digitalcommons.liberty.edu/cgi/viewcontent.cgi?article=1162&context=honors

- https://doi.org/10.1073/pnas.1811878116

- https://doi.org/10.3389%2Ffpsyg.2013.00910

- https://doi.org/10.3389/fpsyg.2013.00910

- https://doi.org/10.3389/fpsyg.2020.01246

- https://doi.org/10.4236/health.2018.109088

- https://pistilsnursery.com/blogs/journal/music-and-plant-growth-heres-what-the-science-says#:~:text=For%20most%20plants%20playing%20classical,they%20prefer%20a%20gentler%20touch.

- https://youtu.be/K3eveCJu_eE

- https://youtu.be/NXCTeo2nMn8

- Keep Your Brain Young with Music | Johns Hopkins Medicine

- Music and the Brain [Effects of Music on the Brain] - Thrive Global

- Neuroscientists Uncover Why the Brain Enjoys Music (scitechdaily.com)

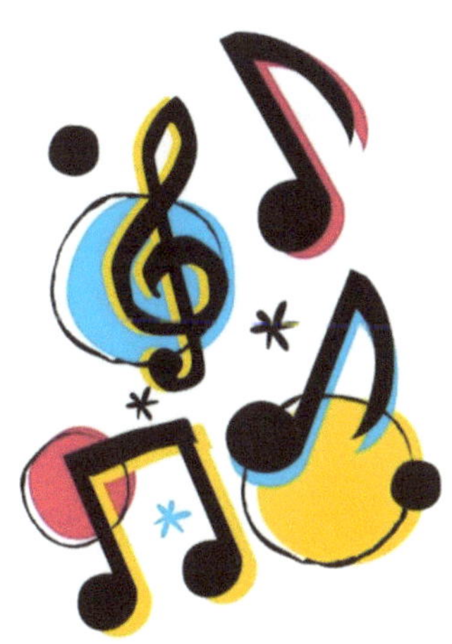

We should not turn the divine

creation of *MUSIC* into **NOISE**

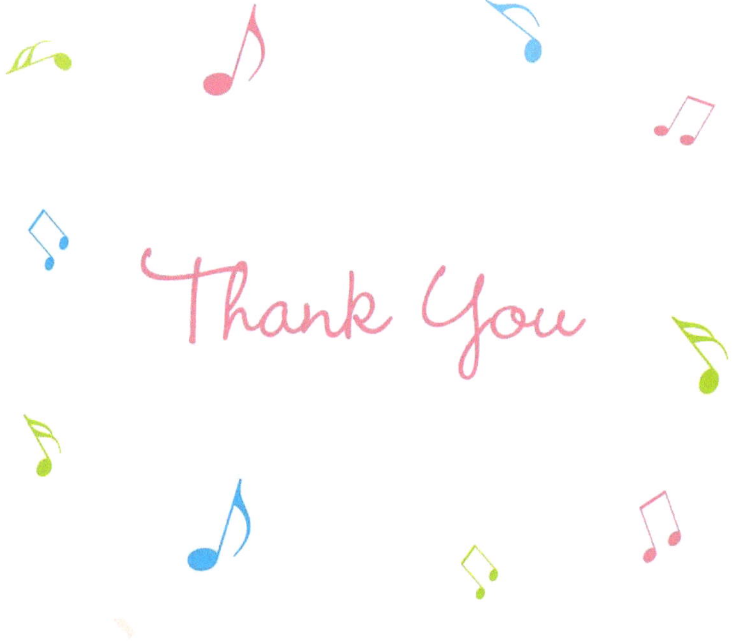